Medical Records
Journal

Medical Records Journal

by

Mary Ann S. Tassey

To order additional copies of this book, contact:
Xlibris Corporation
1-888-795-4274
www.Xlibris.com
Orders@Xlibris.com
129021

TABLE OF CONTENTS

In no way and at no time should this "Medical Records Journal" replace your own personal doctors' medical records and expert advice.

Everyone person is an individualist and no person has all the same physical problems as another.

This Medical Records Journal is mainly for your own personal medical recordkeeping.

It is advised that you always consult your doctor to find out what treatments and tests will best benefit you.

INTRODUCTION

The MEDICAL RECORDS JOURNAL was created so that everyone may keep his or her medical records and appointments together. This will help in assisting you and all of your family in keeping organized medical records. Take your Journal with you to your doctor and decide together which tests are right for you and how often they should be done. Each time you get a test, write the date and the results in your Journal. The more aggressive you are in getting your screenings done as scheduled and recommended by your doctor, in addition to your regular check-ups, the sooner you are going to detect disease and illness in its beginning stages. Prevention remains the most important tool we have in the fight against disease, especially the top three killers of Americans today: heart disease, cancer, and stroke. A Calendar is also provided for all of your appointments.

Under the "NOTES" of the specialty Doctors' Section, list your medications, dosages, pharmacist, possibly a recommended second opinion of a diagnosis, or any other information that may be important to your health. Due to the importance of your medical record-keeping, it is my desire that a copy of this Journal reaches the hands of every person, young and old alike.

Best wishes to you and yours for good health always, and may you live your life to the fullest.

Mary Ann Tassey

DEDICATION

I wish to dedicate this Journal to my beloved sister, Rose, who passed away from breast cancer and who held a very special place in my heart. She was like a second mother to my seven children.

Being a young mother while the children were growing up, I couldn't do it without her and our Heavenly Father.

ACKNOWLEDGEMENTS

I would like to thank my seven wonderful and precious children for their encouragement and help; Michelle Craig, Rachelle Sidone, Richard Hvizdak, Jacque' Daigle. To Mark and Robert Hvizdak for the many hours they put in on the computer due to my many deletions and additions, and last but not least, to Cynthia Rooney, for the valued time she took away from her three little ones, James Gannon, 16 years, Connan Padraig, 14 years, and Muirinn, 10 years, in order to help me with all the research and assistance. Finally, I could never forget to thank all of my friends and relatives, especially those who offered positive advice and support, and to my loving husband, Louis Tassey, who gave me his undivided attention because he, too, realized the importance of my work.

Thanks again to all.

Mary Ann Tassey

KEEPING PHYSICALLY FIT
AND
GENERAL NUTRITION

Many of you are concerned, curious, and sometimes confused about associating nutrition with cancer. Based on evidence at hand, you may lessen your chances of getting cancer by following these simple guidelines:

1. *Avoid obesity.* Being overweight increases the risk of cancer. The American Cancer Society found that obesity was associated with mortality from cancers of the uterus, gallbladder, kidney, stomach, colon, breast, and other organs.

2. *Cut down on total fat and sugar intake.* A high fat and sugar diet increases the risk of developing cancers of the breast, colon, and prostate. The American Cancer Society recommends a daily intake of fat of 30% or less of total calories consumed.

3. *Include a variety of vegetables and fruits in the daily diet.* Dark green and deep yellow vegetables and certain fruits are rich in beta-carotene, a form of vitamin A. People with diets rich in vitamin C are less likely to get cancer, particularly cancer of the stomach and esophagus. Vegetables and fruits are principal sources of vitamin C.

4. *Eat more high-fiber foods* such as whole grain cereals, bread, pastas, vegetables, and fruits.

5. *Limit consumption of alcoholic beverages.* Heavy drinkers of alcohol, especially those who are also cigarette smokers, are at unusually high risk for cancers of the lungs, oral cavity, larynx, and esophagus.

6. *Limit consumption of salt-cured, smoked, and nitrate-cured foods.*

7. *Essential fatty acids (mono and polyunsaturated) are essential for normal and healthy blood vessels.*

8. *Eating several mini meals a day* was cited as one of the top strategies for maintaining a healthy weight.

Remember, weight control, proper eating, and use of supplements are all parts of nutrition.

CANCER

What is cancer? Cancer is a number of diseases caused by the abnormal growth of cells. Normally, the cells that make up the body divide and reproduce in an orderly manner so that you can grow, replace worn out tissue, and repair any injuries. However, when cells grow out of control, they divide more than they should and form masses known as tumors. Some tumors do not spread to other parts of the body but interfere with normal body functions and require removal. These are known as benign tumors. In malignant or cancerous tumors, cells break away from the original tumor and migrate to other parts of the body.

BREAST CANCER:

Breast cancer most often begins as a painless lump or thickening in the upper outer portion of the breast, although it can occur anywhere in the breast. Breast cancers may spread to lymph nodes in the armpits and then through the lymph nodes to the lungs, liver, bone, and brain. The survival rates for breast cancer patients depends on the size of the tumor when first diagnosed. For women with cancer only in the breast, the relative five-year survival rate has increased from 78 percent in the 1940s, to 92 percent today. If, however, the cancer has spread to the region around the breast, the five-year survival rate is 71 percent. For persons with more widespread cancer, the survival rate is 18 percent.

Who is at risk? If you enter menopause at the age of 50 or older, are overweight (postmenopausal), have a first child at 30 or older, have a family history of breast cancer (in a mother, daughter, or sister), or are diagnosed with benign breast disease.

Guidelines for breast cancer detection:

- If you are 20 or over, do a breast self-exam every month.
- In addition to the BSE, if you are 20 to 40, have a clinical breast exam done every three years.
- If you are 40 to 49, have a mammogram done every one to two years.
- If you are 50 or over, schedule a mammogram every year.

NOTE: These guidelines are for women who have no symptoms.

PROSTATE CANCER:
Prostate cancer is the most common cancer in American men. More than 80 percent of prostate cancer cases occur in men age 65 and over.

Who is at risk? If there is a family history, have a diet high in saturated fat or red meat, are increasing in age, and of African American heritage.

LUNG CANCER:
Lung cancer is the leading cancer killer of women. Approximately 59,000 women die each year of lung cancer, while 46,000 women die each year of breast cancer, according to the American Cancer Society.

Who is at risk? If you are a cigarette smoker, take in secondhand smoke, are increasing in age, and have a diet low in fruits and vegetables.

UTERINE CANCER:
Uterine cancer can strike a woman at any age; however, fewer women die from cancer of the uterus each year because they have regular pap smear tests.

Who is at risk? If you are over 40, overweight, taking hormone treatment, have abnormal bleeding, are infertile, or do not ovulate.

COLON AND RECTAL CANCER:
Third major cancer killer in women and most often strikes women over age 50.

Who is at risk? If you have a family member with colon or rectal cancer, are increasing in age, Jewish (European Heritage), have a diet high in saturated fat or red meat and low in fruits, vegetables, whole grain, and beans.

HEART DISEASE

While heart disease is the leading cause of death in the United States among men and women, remember you have the power to help reduce your risk. By eating well, exercising, and not smoking, you can be well on your way to a heart-healthy lifestyle. Studies from all over the world have shown a link between a high fat diet and an increased risk of premature death from heart attack.

- Heart attack, stroke, and other cardiovascular diseases have killed more women than men every year since 1984.
- Arteriosclerosis, a progressive, destructive, thickening of blood vessels due to fat and cholesterol plaques is the direct result of excessive carbohydrates. Arteriosclerosis results in fatal heart disease, high blood pressure, brain damage (strokes and senility), aneurysms, and other diseases which cause more than twice as many deaths each year in the United States as all cancers combined.
- More than one out of five women has some form of cardiovascular disease. (This was unheard of years ago in women.)
- Cardiovascular diseases kill more women than all forms of cancer, chronic lung disease, pneumonia, diabetes, accidents, and A.I.D.S combined.
- One in every three women will die of coronary heart disease or heart attack.

Premenopausal women rarely get heart disease because their own estrogen naturally protects them. This essential hormone helps keep total blood cholesterol low. Before the age of 45, most women have cholesterol counts within the acceptable range of 185 to 200.

Who is at risk? If you are premenopausal, your own estrogen protects you from heart disease. If any of the following applies to you, you are considered at risk:

- If you smoke.
- If you have a family history of premature heart disease.
- If you are over 54, or going through premature menopause.
- If you do not exercise.
- If you have diabetes or high blood pressure.
- If you are obese.
- If your HDL is below 35.

If you have high blood pressure, your risk of having a heart attack increases by 210 percent.

According to studies, aspirin helps keep blood from clotting and reduces your chance of another heart attack. If you do have a heart attack, it is likely to be less severe. However, check with your doctor if you have liver or kidney disease, an ulcer, or high blood pressure before taking aspirin. Some symptoms of a heart attack include heavy sweating, shortness of breath, crushing or squeezing chest pain, dizziness, and nausea or vomiting.

CHOLESTEROL & TRIGLYCERIDES

What is cholesterol? In order to help build cells, your body uses cholesterol, a fatty substance found in your blood. Your own liver manufactures all the cholesterol you need. Why is it so bad for you? Many of us eat too much of it. The excess cholesterol your body does not need is deposited in your blood vessels in the form of bumps called plaque. As plaque builds up, your blood vessels harden and narrow, making your heart work harder. Plaque deposits can cause blood clots that can completely block blood flow which may eventually result in a heart attack or stroke. If you ate nothing at all, the body would continue to manufacture cholesterol. Your body needs a certain amount of cholesterol. More than half of the people in the United States do not know their cholesterol level. Do you know your cholesterol numbers? There are two types of cholesterol: low-density lipoprotein (LDL) and high-density lipoprotein (HDL). An excess of LDL buildup in the blood vessels hinders the flow of blood. LDL is also known as "bad" cholesterol. Your LDL level is high if it is160 mg/dl or above. Borderline is 130 to 159 mg/dl. The ideal is lower than 130 mg/dl. Note: If you or your immediate family have heart disease, the LDL, "bad" cholesterol should be under 100. If your LDL is too high, cut your saturated fats to 10% of total calories. If that does not work, then cut them to 7%. If your LDL level stays high despite dietary changes, you may need medication. HDL, or "good" cholesterol, is believed to help clear blood vessels by carrying cholesterol back to the liver. The average person should maintain a total cholesterol level below 200 mg/dl. People with otherwise normal total cholesterol levels of 200 mg/dl or less can still have a heart attack. Your HDL is definitely too low if it is below 35 mg/dl, "and for women, anything below 45 mg/dl may be risky", says Angelo M. Scanu, M.D., Director of the Lipoprotein Study Unit at the University of Chicago

School of Medicine. The ideal is to have an HDL count of 60 mg/dl or above. The average American man consumes about 450 mgs of cholesterol per day; the average woman, about 320 mgs. The American Heart Association recommends a daily in-take of cholesterol of below 300 mgs.

The key to lower cholesterol levels is to reduce your intake of cholesterol and saturated fat. Avoid foods that are high in saturated fat such as solid shortening and palm and coconut oils.
Use monounsaturated (canola, olive, peanut) oils when cooking.

Who is at risk? If you are a man 45 years old or older, or a woman 55 years old or older, have a family history of heart problems or heart disease, have high blood pressure, smoke, are a woman who has gone through early menopause and are not taking estrogen replacement therapy, and if you have diabetes.

Triglycerides: Normal levels pose risks too. Carbohydrates and dietary fats are converted to blood fats called Triglycerides. Once considered relatively innocent, a high triglycerides level has now been shown to greatly increase heart disease risk. A triglyceride level of 400 mg/dl or above is dangerously high. A reading of 200 to 399 mg/dl is borderline. The ideal is under 100 mg/dl. Traditionally, any reading below 200 was considered desirable, but a recent study discovered that people with triglyceride levels greater than 100 mg/dl had twice as many heart attacks as those who had lower triglyceride levels. If your number is too high, replace saturated fat with omega-3 fatty acids found in salmon and other fatty fish. "Avoid alcohol if your triglyceride level is over 200", says Michael Miller, M.D., Director of Preventive Cardiology at the University of Maryland School of Medicine.

CHANGING YOUR DIET FOR YOUR HEART:

Changes in your diet can lower your risk factors for heart disease. Make sure your diet is low in fat especially saturated fat, cholesterol, sugar and sodium, and high in dietary fiber and complex carbohydrates.

Diets high in oatmeal or oat bran and low in saturated fat and cholesterol may reduce the risk of heart disease. Oats lower both total cholesterol and LDL cholesterol. Experts believe oat soluble fiber reduces cholesterol.

BLOOD PRESSURE

When your blood pressure is too high, your heart has to work harder to pump blood through your body. The natural force created when your heart pumps blood into your blood vessels is known as blood pressure. For a variety of reasons, your blood vessels can tighten and constrict. This can cause the blood to press on the vessel walls with too much force. When the force remains above a certain level, it is considered high blood pressure. Being overweight is one of the most common health risks for Americans today. In combination with high blood pressure, being overweight can contribute to increased risk of heart disease. Limit fat intake to less than 30% of your total daily calories, limit daily cholesterol intake to less than 300 milligrams, and limit egg yolk, organ meats, animal fats, and whole milk products. Eat more fruits, vegetables, whole grains, lean meats, and skinless chicken. Try to fit a daily walk into your routine.

What you can do to reduce your risk factors:
Whatever your risk factors, you'll lower your chances of developing heart disease if you:

- Exercise for at least 30 minutes three or four times a week.
- Maintain a healthy weight.
- Cut saturated fat (avoid red meat and high-fat dairy products) and trans fats found in margarine and processed foods made with partially hydrogenated oils.
- Do not smoke. If you quit now, you can lower your heart attack risk by 50 percent in one year.
- Have your blood pressure checked regularly by your doctor.

CHOOSING FOOD TO REACH YOUR GOAL:

Shopping for the right foods does not have to be confusing or overwhelming. With a little practice, you can develop skills for reducing fats by reading labels, and making good selections at the store.

- Pick your fats wisely. Your goals are to choose less saturated fat and to eat less fat overall. Use small portions of monounsaturated and polyunsaturated fats instead of saturated fat. Avoid saturated fat from animal sources such as butter, lard, and fatty meats. Vegetable sources are coconut, palm, and "partially hydrogenated" oils which are found in many processed foods. Double check labels that boast "no cholesterol", and avoid a product in which coconut or palm oil or hydrogenated vegetable shortening are among the first ingredients listed.

- Experiments have proven that eating trans fatty acids produce harmful changes in blood cholesterol levels, and studies demonstrate that people who eat more trans fats get more heart attacks. Women who consumed the most trans fatty acids had one and one-half times more heart attacks than women who consumed the least trans fat did. The increased risk was linked to partially hydrogenated vegetable oils, margarine, and other foods that contain vegetable shortening, including cookies, cake, and white bread.

READ THE LABELS

The best way to find fats and cholesterol in processed foods is to read the labels. Ideally, less than 30 percent of your day's total calories should come from fat. However, if you wish to lose weight, it should be 20 percent or less. If fat is a major ingredient, the product contains too much fat.

GUIDELINES FOR A HEALTHY DIET:

1. Keep fat intake to less than or equal to 30 percent of your total daily calories.
2. Limit saturated fat to 8 percent to 10 percent of total daily calories.
3. Lower cholesterol intake to less than 300 mgs per day.
4. Choose foods high in starch and fiber.
5. Read the labels to find the nutritional value.

FOOD CHAIN PYRAMID

The food chain pyramid is an outline of what to eat each day based on the dietary guidelines. A guide helps you choose a healthful diet that is right for you, and at the same time, chooses the right amount of calories to maintain a healthy weight. There are several dietary guidelines that can help you improve your health and reduce your chances of getting certain diseases such as high blood pressure, heart disease, strokes, and certain cancers. The guidelines are as follows:

Maintain a healthy weight.

- Choose a diet low in fat, saturated fat, and cholesterol.
- Choose a diet with plenty of vegetables, fruits, and grain products.
- Use sugars and salts in moderation.

The food chain pyramid is as follows:

- ☑ 6 to 11   Bread, cereal, rice and pasta group
- ☑ 3 to 5   Vegetable group
- ☑ 2 to 4   Fruit group
- ☑ 2 to 3   Dairy group (milk, yogurt and cheese)
- ☑ 2 to 3   Meat, poultry and fish
- ☑ In Moderation   Fats, oils and sweets

The number of servings that are right for you depends on how many calories you need which, in turn, depends on your age, sex, size, and how active you are. Almost everyone should have at least the lowest number of servings in the ranges.

METABOLISM

The rate at which your body burns calories when it is at rest plays an important part in determining your body weight. The slower your metabolism, the fewer calories you burn, and the more difficulty you will have controlling your weight. If you are overweight, your resting metabolic rate may be lower than that of normal-weight people. The average adult gets about 37 percent of total calories from fat. Regular physical activity causes several changes in your body and has a positive impact on your weight-regulating system. As you lose weight, your body's weight regulator will start to gear down your metabolism to make up for your lighter weight and your lower caloric intake. This will cause you to burn slightly fewer calories each day. Females beginning to push forty experience a double whammy: metabolic slowdown calling for fewer calories and hormonal changes calling for tighter control of carbohydrate intake. While most of today's weight-loss diets control calories, they tend to be high in carbohydrates. They fail to address the hormonal changes that make this group of women fail on such diets. A low fat, high-fiber diet is recommended by the American Cancer Society, the American Heart Association, and the American Diabetes Association because high-fiber foods are generally low fat and calorie-light, puffed up by nature with a healthy proportion of indigestible bulk. This bulk satisfies the need to chew and fills the stomach, but it leaves the body without being metabolized or storing unwanted body fat.

VITAMIN RECOMMENDATIONS

- Vitamin A (beta carotene): Beta-carotene is converted in the body to vitamin A, essential for good immunity. Low levels predict high levels of cancer, heart disease and infections.

  Some examples are carrots, green and yellow vegetables, milk and dairy products, yellow fruits, eggs, and liver. If your daily diet includes ample amounts of the above, it is unlikely you need an A supplement.

- Vitamin B6: Lack of B6 is linked to increased heart attacks, strokes, and depression. It works as a natural diuretic. If you are on the pill, you are more than likely to need increased amounts of B6.

  Some examples are wheat bran, wheat germ, cabbage, cantaloupe, spinach, fresh tuna, broccoli, eggs and milk.

- Vitamin B12: Critical in maintaining normal brain and nervous system functioning. What it can do for you is form and regenerate red blood cells, thereby preventing anemia. It also increases energy, improves concentration, memory and balance.

  Some examples are liver, beef, pork, eggs, milk and cheeses.

- Vitamin C: A strong anti-oxidant. Deficiency is linked to increased colds and infections, cancer, heart disease, high blood pressure, asthma and high blood cholesterol. Some examples are citrus fruits, berries, green and leafy vegetables, tomatoes, cauliflower, potatoes and broccoli.

- Vitamin E: Another anti-oxidant that keeps arteries clear by blocking toxic changes in bad type LDL cholesterol so it cannot invade artery walls and accumulate debris or plaque. What it can do for you is supply oxygen to the body to give you more endurance, protect your lungs against air pollution by working with vitamin A, prevents and dissolves blood clots, and it works as a diuretic which can lower blood pressure.

  Some examples are wheat germ, vegetable oils, broccoli, brussel sprouts, leafy greens, whole grain cereals and eggs.

- Calcium: A well-known protector of bones, it is also tied to lessen high blood pressure and colon cancer. Eating calcium rich foods helps maximize bone mass, warding off crippling osteoporosis in later life. What it can do for you is maintain strong bones and healthy teeth, keep your heart beating regularly and metabolize your body's iron.

  Some examples are milk and milk products, all cheeses, sardines, walnuts, sunflower seeds, and green vegetables.

- Potassium: Works with sodium to regulate the body's water balance and normalize heart rhythms. It also helps normalize blood pressure. What it can do for you is help dispose of body wastes, assist in reducing blood pressure and aids in clear thinking by sending oxygen to the brain.

  Some examples are citrus fruits, green leafy vegetables, sunflower seeds, bananas and potatoes.

- Folic acid: Helps fight heart disease, strokes, cancer, depression, and loss of mental acuity. It is crucial in fighting artery clogging homocysteine (an amino acid that is a potent emerging risk factor for heart disease). A high level of homocysteine triples your chance of having a heart attack. It also aids in protein metabolism. What it can do for you is protects against intestinal parasites and food poisoning, improves lactation and helps ward off anemia.

Some examples are deep green leafy vegetables, carrots, egg yolk, cantaloupe, apricots, whole wheat and dark rye flour.

- Zinc: Helps in the formation of insulin which is important for blood stability and in maintaining the body's acid-alkaline balance, exerts a normalizing effect on the prostate and is important in the development of all reproductive organs. It can promote growth and mental alertness, help to decrease cholesterol deposits and helps avoid prostate problems.

Some examples are wheat germ, pumpkin seeds, eggs, lean beef, spinach and nonfat dry milk.

- Magnesium: Protects against heart disease, high blood pressure and diabetes. It is important for converting blood sugar into energy and is essential for effective nerve and muscle functioning. What it can do for you is promote a healthier cardiovascular system and help prevent heart attacks; it also helps prevent calcium deposits, kidney and gallstones and aids in fighting depression.

Some examples are figs, lemons, grapefruit, almonds, nuts, dark green vegetables, apples, wheat bran and spinach.

CARDIOLOGIST

Doctor: _____

Address: _____

_____

Phone Number: _____

Fax Number: _____

TYPE OF TESTING	DATE of TESTING	LOCATION OF TESTING	RESULTS
Blood Pressure			
EKG			
Ultrasound			
Cholesterol Check			
Flu Shot			
Pneumonia Shot			

General Notes For Testing:

MEDICATIONS:

PRESCRIPTION	DATE PRESCRIBED	DOSAGE

FAMILY PRACTIONER

Doctor: _____

Address: _____

_____

Phone Number: _____

Fax Number: _____

TYPE OF TESTING	DATE of TESTING	LOCATION OF TESTING	RESULTS
Blood Pressure			
Screening			
X-Ray			
Tetanus-Deptheria			
Shot			
Blood Work			
Cholesterol Check			
Flu Shot			
Pneumonia Shot			
Lipid Profile			
Bone Density			
Skin Cancer			
Screening			
Colonoscopy			
Allergies			

General Notes For Testing:

MEDICATIONS:

PRESCRIPTION	DATE PRESCRIBED	DOSAGE

GYNECOLOGIST

Doctor: _____

Address: _____

_____

Phone Number: _____

Fax Number: _____

TYPE OF TESTING	DATE of TESTING	LOCATION OF TESTING	RESULTS

General Notes For Testing:

MEDICATIONS:

PRESCRIPTION	DATE PRESCRIBED	DOSAGE

NEUROLOGIST

Doctor: _____

Address: _____

_____

Phone Number: _____

Fax Number: _____

TYPE OF TESTING	DATE of TESTING	LOCATION OF TESTING	RESULTS
Cat Scan			
X-Ray			
Radioisotope Scan			
MRI			

General Notes For Testing:

MEDICATIONS:

PRESCRIPTION	DATE PRESCRIBED	DOSAGE

ONCOLOGIST

Doctor: _____

Address: _____

_____

Phone Number: _____

Fax Number: _____

TYPE OF TESTING	DATE of TESTING	LOCATION OF TESTING	RESULTS
Cat Scan			
Chemotherapy			
Radiation Therapy			
Biopsy			
Blood Test			

General Notes For Testing:

MEDICATIONS:

PRESCRIPTION	DATE PRESCRIBED	DOSAGE

OPHTHALMOLOGIST

Doctor: _____

Address: _____

_____

Phone Number: _____

Fax Number: _____

TYPE OF TESTING	DATE of TESTING	LOCATION OF TESTING	RESULTS
Vision Exam			
Glaucoma Exam			
Cataract			
Infection			

General Notes For Testing:

MEDICATIONS:

PRESCRIPTION	DATE PRESCRIBED	DOSAGE

ORTHOPEDIC

Doctor:

Address:

Phone Number:

Fax Number:

TYPE OF TESTING	DATE of TESTING	LOCATION OF TESTING	RESULTS
X-Ray			
Bone Scan			
Blood Test			
CAT Scan			

General Notes For Testing:

MEDICATIONS:

PRESCRIPTION	DATE PRESCRIBED	DOSAGE

PEDIATRICIAN

Doctor: _____

Address: _____

_____

Phone Number: _____

Fax Number: _____

Child's Age	Type of Immunization	Date of Shot	Location
Birth	- Hepatitis B		
	-		
	-		
2 months	- 2nd Hepatitis B		
	- DTP (Diphtheria, Tetanus, Pertussis)		
	- H Influenza type B (hib)		
	- Polio (IPV or OPV)		
	-		
4 months	- 2nd DTP		
	- 2nd Hib		
	- 2nd Polio		
	-		
6 months	- 3rd Hepatitis B		
	- 3rd DTP		
	- 3rd Hib		
	- 3rd Polio		
	-		
	-		
12 months	- 4th DTP		
	- Final Hib		

Child's Age	Type of Immunization	Date of Shot	Location
12 months	- MMR (Measles, Mumps, Rubella)		
	- VZV (Chicken Pox Vaccine)		
	-		
18 months	-		
	-		
	-		
	-		
24 months	-		
	-		
	-		
	-		
	-		
4 to 6 yrs	- 5th DTP		
	- 4th Polio		
	- 2nd MMR (Measles, Mumps, Rubella)		
11 to 12 yrs	- TD (Tetanus, Diphtheria) (If 5 years since last DTP shot.)		
	-		
	-		
	-		

General Notes For Immunization:

MEDICATIONS:

PRESCRIPTION	DATE PRESCRIBED	DOSAGE

UROLOGIST

Doctor: _____

Address: _____

_____

Phone Number: _____

Fax Number: _____

TYPE OF TESTING	DATE of TESTING	LOCATION OF TESTING	RESULTS
Prostate Exam			
PSA (Prostate			
specific Antigen)			
Blood Test			
Urine Test			

General Notes For Testing:

MEDICATIONS:

PRESCRIPTION	*DATE PRESCRIBED*	*DOSAGE*

PHYSICIAN

Doctor: _____

Address: _____

_____

Phone Number: _____

Fax Number: _____

TYPE OF TESTING	DATE of TESTING	LOCATION OF TESTING	RESULTS

General Notes For Testing:

MEDICATIONS:

PRESCRIPTION	DATE PRESCRIBED	DOSAGE

PHARMACY

Pharmacy Name: _____
Pharmacist: _____
Address: _____
_____

Phone Number: _____
Fax Number: _____

PRESCRIPTION	DATE PRESCRIBED	DOSAGE

General Pharmacy Notes:

General Notes:

www.ingramcontent.com/pod-product-compliance
Lightning Source LLC
Chambersburg PA
CBHW021915170526
45157CB00005B/2079